Nursing Mnemonics:

The Ultimate Tips and Notes For Nurses

By

Brittany Samons

Table of Contents

Nursing Mnemonics: The Ultimate Tips and Notes For Nurses

By Brittany Samons

Introduction

As a nurse, you always need to have the right answers to a problem at the right time. You can never make any mistakes, or the time to peruse through books seeking for clarification. With so much to cram into your head, mastering disease conditions and their treatment options is quite the challenge. Taking a different approach other than just trying to remember the facts as they are would make the job simpler and more bearable. Enter mnemonics.

A mnemonic is a Greek word that literally translates to 'memory aid.' A good mnemonic ought to be a simple easy to remember phrase whose letters stand for a specific term. Once you have this phrase in mind, all you need is a hazy idea of the specific terms it stands for. After this, all you will ever have to do is remember the mnemonic and use its letters to guide your brain into remembering the exact fact you are looking for. Here are useful and perhaps the easiest to remember mnemonics that will make your nursing career simpler.

Part 1. Cardiovascular Acronyms

1 Myocardial Infarction (heart attack)

Heart attacks need immediate attention to prevent fatal heart damage that could lead to death. The MONA acronym is a perfect way to remember what you need to handle heart attacks.

Morphine: To alleviate the chest pain that accompanies the heart attack

Oxygen: A continuous supply of pure oxygen will prevent hypoxia to offset the inadequacy.

Nitroglycerin: Lowers blood pressure and reduces heart's demand for oxygen.

Aspirin: Used to dissolve the blood clot that led to the heart attack.

For better remembrance, rearrange the acronym to ONAM and use 'I am ON fire in the AM as I am a morning person.'

Remember that acting fast and right could be the only thing between you and your patient's life. Knowing your tools and having them nearby at all times will help you handle such a situation better.

2 Congestive Heart Failure

This condition will happen when the heart cannot keep up with the high blood output in the circulatory system. The acronym UNLOAD FAST should guide you through the management process.

Upright: Keep the patient in an upright position

Nitrates: Use a nitrate, for instance Nitroglycerin to cut down on the heart's oxygen demand

Lasix: Facilitates fluid loss from blood through diuresis hence reducing blood volume

Oxygen: supply of pure oxygen to keep the body functional during the temporal heart failure

ACE Inhibitors: encourage vasodilation to accommodate the increased blood volume.

Digoxin: Reduces the ventricular rate

The second part of the acronym is all about limiting and reducing factors that could reverse what you have already done. These are:

Fluids: decrease on fluid intake

Afterload: the decrease in fluid intake and getting rid of excess fluid contributes to reducing the afterload.

Sodium: Sodium restriction is important since more sodium in the body will encourage the kidney to reabsorb fluids back into the blood.

Test: Finally, do continuous tests to monitor the patient's condition

Inasmuch as everything you do helps the patient to recover, there are a couple of things you constantly monitor to ensure everything is going on as expected. An overdose of digoxin is toxic. You must keep the dosage in check. Monitoring the ABGs will ensure that you provide the right oxygen levels to the patient's blood while a frequent serum potassium test will help you keep fluid volume excess in check.

3 Lead II Placement

Good electrode placement will determine the accuracy of the EKG strips obtained. Even though there are other things to consider when doing the lead II placement, the most common is the orientation of the electrodes. The SALT, PEPPER, KETCHUP acronym will help.

Salt: the white electrode comes first (start from your upper left, the patients upper right)

Pepper: the black electrode on the opposite side of the white

Ketchup: The red electrode should be placed over the heart (the patient's lower left chest). If you have done the orientation right, it will be below the black electrode.

Ensure that you remove any hair at the point where the electrode makes contact with the skin by using an electric clipper since razors will abrade and irritate the skin. Before applying the electrodes, rub the area with an alcohol swatch and ensure that the electrodes have a fair share or gel.

4 Angina Precipitation Factors: 4 E's

Angina is a chest pain that arises from reduced blood flow to your heart. It is an onset to heart conditions and should get treated immediately after it is detected. The factors to consider when diagnosing it include:

Exertion: Extremely tired or feels the pain more after exercise or physical activity

Eating: Has difficulties when eating or loss of appetite.

Emotional distress: Is stressed up and not emotionally stable.

Extreme temperatures: very hot or cold weather could trigger it.

Symptoms can always mean another health condition. Piecing up the basic Angina symptoms and combining them with tests is crucial to identifying this problem.

5 Blood Pressure: BP = CO x SVR

Taking a patient's blood pressure is a normal everyday activity. Here is a simple formula that will help you remember how it is done.

Blood **P**ressure

Cardiac **O**utput

Systemic **V**ascular **R**esistance

There is a wide variety of tools used to take these basic readings needed to calculate blood pressure. Learn how to use the most common tools available in your market.

6 Leukemia Symptoms

Leukemia is all about the white blood cells. They could insufficient, immature or malformed. The ANT acronym will help you identify the basic symptoms of Leukemia.

A: Anemia that is characterized by a drop in HGM count drop

N: Neutropenia, this is an increased risk of infection since white blood cells don't work optimally

T: Thrombocytopenia leading to excessing bleeding

Think of it as a huge number of immature ants, they will be white hence, it will bring the relation you need to remember the acronym and what it stands for.

7 Intensive care patient management

This is aimed at giving patients at the intensive care better systematic care hence increasing their rate of recovery. The mnemonic to use here is 'give your patient a FAST HUG'

Feeding: Ensure that the patient is well fed at regular intervals.

Analgesia: Use of painkiller to alleviate pain will keep the patient more comfortable.

Sedation: If the condition is to serious, sedation or an induced comma will help.

Thromboembolic prophylaxis: If the patient has this condition, take great care to address it.

Head-of-bed elevation: keeping the head slightly elevated aids in blood circulation and respiration.

Stress Ulcer prevention: staying in one position for long could lead to stress ulcers. Change positions often.

Glucose control: Blood sugar level is important for strength and normal bodily function.

This simple technique can be done anytime to all patients in the intensive care unit. It is not mandatory. It will however improve on the quality of care you give at the ICU.

8 Hypoglycemia Causes and Characteristics

Mnemonic: RE-EXPLAIN

Renal failure: This is when the kidney cannot get rid of the wastes in blood making them pile up.

Exogenous: external factors that could lead to the symptoms and problems related to hypoglycemia.

Pituitary: The pituitary is overworked and might exhibit some problems

Liver failure: The liver fails to handle insulin production and general blood sugar regulation.

Alcohol use: frequent alcohol use could lead to liver and renal failure.

Infections: frequent infections arising from the multiple organ failures.

Neoplasm: This abnormal tissue growth could affect the epithelial cells.

Hypoglycemia is best diagnosed by using its symptoms and the patient's behaviors. Creating a link between the existing symptoms and lifestyle will help you identify whether the symptoms point to this conditions. Have a good chat with the patient to get all the facts you need.

9 Hypernatremia signs and symptoms

Mnemonic: FRIED

Flushed skin and low grade fever

Restless, irritability, anxiousness, confusion

Increased blood pressure and fluid retention

Edema: peripheral and pitting

Decreased urine output and dry mouth

Some of the symptoms like blood pressure can be identified by running a simple test. A better part of the symptoms and signs are only visible if you talk to the patient. Establishing a good rapport and taking the patient through an aided question and answer session will help you identify these signs in the most friendly way possible.

10 Hypernatremia Causes: MODEL

Meals (high intake) and medications that could contribute to higher concentrations of sodium in the body.

Osmotic diuresis: Increased urination due to the presence of some substances in kidneys that cannot be reabsorbed into the body.

Diabetes Insipidus: Excessive thirst and passing of a lot of dilute urine meaning that the body is not doing excretion via urine well.

Excessive loss of water: Loosing a lot of water mostly via passing a lot of dilute urine.

Low intake of water: Though rare, the condition could also arise from not taking sufficient amounts of water in a day.

This condition is directly linked to dehydration. Helping your patient recover the lost water before treating he condition causing the loss is key to handling the condition completely. Remember that loss of water that increases the sodium levels hence increasing water levels, rather than reducing sodium levels, is the right treatment.

11 Hypocalcaemia Signs and Symptoms: CATS

Convulsions: Involuntary contraction and relaxation of muscles making limbs move around uncontrollably.

Arrhythmias: irregular heart beat arising from the convulsions.

Tetany: This is another word for seizures. It is an indicator of involuntary muscle movement.

Stridor and spasms: This will occur when the involuntary muscle contraction is at a lower level.

This condition relates to serum calcium levels. Since cellular processes regulate calcium levels in the body, the condition should indicate some problem in these processes. The deficiency should be used to diagnose these conditions.

Part 2. Hyperkalemia

Hyperkalemia is a condition related to high potassium concentration in the blood. Since potassium is an electrolyte, its concentration in the body is visible after doing an electrocardiography. Since the symptoms are non-specific, the condition is normally detected in a blood test run for another reason. Handling it in time is crucial since when it moves on; it could lead to arrhythmia (abnormal heart rhythm.)

12 Hyperkalemia Causes: MACHINE

Medicine: the NSAIDS, the ACE inhibitors lastly the Diuretics or the potassium sparing. When administering these three kind dugs to people you may suffer from hyperkalemia.

Acidosis: metabolic and respiratory

Destruction of the Cellular; traumatic injury or even burns and any damage to body cells due to different forms of injury

And in the blood which undergo the hemolysis and Hypoaldosteronism.

Intake: large amount of potassium intake like for example the replacement of salt in your body which has potassium content.

Nephrons: will lead to failure of your renal

Excretion: faulty or impaired excretion process

13 Hyperkalemia the Signs and the Symptoms: MURDER

Muscle cramping and it will lead to body weakness.

Urine abnormalities: oliguria or anuria (output less than 30 mL/hour or no output)

Respiratory distress like breathing complications

Decreased cardiac contractility that could contribute to the chest discomfort.

EKG changes

Reflexes: hyperreflexia or areflexia (flaccidity)

14 Hypokalemia Signs and Symptoms: A SIC WALT

Alkalosis: A blood serum pH that is higher than normal (7.45 or higher)

Shallow Respirations: Shallow and fast breathing as if after some form of exertion.

Irritability: Easy to irritate and annoy out of no apparent reason

Confusion and drowsiness: The patient appears tired or rather sleepy and does not have a strong idea of what is going on.

Weakness and fatigue: Weakened patient who appears ever tired and not strong enough.

Arrhythmias: either the bradycardia or tachycardia but both of this is the heart's irregular rhythm

Lethargy: This is a condition characterized by fatigue, feeling drowsy and long sleep patterns.

Thready Pulse: A weak pulse.

Apart from this, this condition also has other symptoms that you should look out for. These include the ileus, the vomiting and the mobility of your intestine are decreased.

15 Hypokalemia Causes and Characteristics: SUCTION

Skeletal muscle weakness that makes the patient feel weak at the limbs

U-wave on the EKG result: its origin is yet on discussion but it is an accompaniment of this condition

Constipation: Hard to pass bowels or inconsistent bowel movement.

Toxicity when digoxin is taken: Digoxin is a drug used to treat congestive heart conditions

Irregular and the weakness of your pulses: This can be picked by a stethoscope or by looking at the EKG

Orthostasis: This condition is common to people suffering from this condition.

Numbness paresthesia: Feeling numb at parts of your limbs and finding hardness in moving them

16 Hypokalemia Signs and Symptoms: 6 L's

Lethargy: Continued fatigue and drowsiness.

Leg cramps: Pain in the leg and difficulty in moving your leg muscles

Limp muscles: Non-responsive muscles, especially muscles controlled voluntarily.

Low, shallow respirations: laboured breathing as if the patient is falling short of breath

Lethal cardiac dysrhythmias: Also known as irregular heartbeat and can also constitute of too slow or too fast heartbeat.

Lots of urine (polyuria): Excessive passing of urine, mostly dilute urine.

Even though temporary treatment can alleviate all the hyperkalemia symptoms and create a new balance of the potassium ions, sometimes it is necessary to stimulate urine production by doing dialysis. Making the treatment gradual will help you use the most efficient condition possible.

Part 3. Endocrine System

17 Acute Pancreatitis: GET SMASH'D

Gallstones: Calculus stones formed in the gallbladder as a result of high concentration in bile matter.

Ethanol: A lot of ethanol in the body is harmful to the pancreases.

Trauma: Direct injury to the organ could kick start this condition

Steroids: Excessive use of different types of steroids puts pressure on this and many other body organs

Mumps: This is a viral disease caused by a virus, mumps virus. Its most notable symptom is swelling of the parotid glands.

Autoimmune (PAN): Body reaction to its own blood cells that make it destroy its own cells.

Scorpion bites: scorpion poison is known to induce pancreatitis.

Hyperlipidemia: High concentrations of any or all of the lipids in the blood's serum.

That last D after the apostrophe will tell you the drugs to use in curing the condition.

Drugs such as azathioprine and diuretics

Acute pancreatitis is the sudden inflammation of the pancreases. It could arise from any of the stated conditions in the acronym. Simple cases could be handled by lack of food accompanied by an IV. If the attack is severe, you must refer the patient to surgery to save his or her life.

Part 4. Fundamental Nursing Practices

While you might imagine that your daily nursing life will always be about helping take care of patients, sometimes you are required to either teach them or carry out non-treatment related processes that will help you save life. Here are the most common activities to teach or carry out and the mnemonic like acronyms to help you remember them.

18 Activities of Daily Living (ADLs): BATTED

Bathing: Self hygiene which involves showering and brushing of the teeth

Ambulation: This is another name referring to walking. This refers to the ability to walk properly.

Toileting: Going for short or long calls without the need of any help

Transfers: The ability to move from one place to another with the use of own power or limbs

Eating: Ability to eat food. Sometimes includes the ability to prepare the food itself.

Dressing: Putting on clothes sufficiently and being presentable.

These daily activities, if done well, contribute to healthy life. They are our first defense against diseases. Ensuring that you do them to a patient will get his or her body stronger while boosting their morale. Teaching a patient to do them on his or her own will improve on his health later.

19 Precaution when it comes to bleeding: RANDI

Razor blades as well as the electric blades, keep them away or handle them carefully.

Aspirin inhibits the formation of blood clots. While it is good in clearing heart attach causing clots, it is bad for patients with open wounds.

Needles: Especially the gauges which the sizes are smaller but the diameter are larger lead to more bleeding

Decrease number of needle sticks

Injury risk prevention

Bleeding could be easy to contain. However, in most cases, it is always better to prevent it rather than wait for it to occur and try to prevent it. This acronym furnishes you with the things you need to consider to prevent the bleeding or treat it as soon as possible.

20 Careful Planning: The 3 C's

Collaboration: Talk to the patient and show that you are planning things together.

Cooperation: Show that you are willing to work with the patient

Compromise: Be willing to make trade-offs in your quest to success

This is the most effective preparation for any condition. When dealing with the patient or fellow people, you will have to employ these 3 C's all the way. The help make the chosen path of action more effective and smoother.

21 Hypertension Nursing Interventions: I TIRED!

Intake and output (urine)

Take your blood pressure

Ischemia attack and the transient or known as the TIAs: you should be aware of the signs

Respiration and the monitoring of pulse

Electrolytes: values should be monitor and the blood work should be done by orders

Daily monitoring of weights

22 Instrumental Activities of Daily Living (IADLs): SCUM

Shopping

Cooking

Using the telephone and transportation (driving, public, or ability to independently arrange transportation services)

Money and medication management

An evaluation of the ability to use tools needed to accomplish these activities will help determine whether the patient needs constant care or not.

23 Pain Assessment: PQRST

What Provokes the pain

What is the Quality of the pain?

Does the pain Radiate?

What is the Severity of the pain?

What is the Timing of the pain?

Pain is one of the simplest ways to assessing internal injury or estimating the extent to which a given ailment has spread. Other than helping you prescribe the right treatment, this approach will also help you choose the best way to support the patient in question.

24 Pain Management: ABCDE

Assess for pain and ask about the pain

Believe in whatever description the patient gives to his or her pain known to be the subjective data

Choices: for pain relief, the patients should be aware of

Deliver possible intervention for therapeutic whenever the patient needs it

Empower and enable the pain control on your patient

This acronym comes from the first letters of the alphabet. It is an ideal way to assess the patients pain and it also teaches the importance of taking in the patient's facts as the bare truth. After this, you will know the things to tell the patient and help him handle the pain better.

25 Stool Assessment: FACT

Frequency: How often does it happen?

Amount: how much of it at a time?

Color and consistency: What is its color and general texture?

Timing: at what time does it happen?

Stool assessment should always be done on fresh stool. Encouraging and advising the patient on how to collect the stool right will ensure that it does not get contaminated in the process.

Part 5. Hepatic Related Mnemonics

26 Home Health Nursing Manager: CAME

Clinician: Help with the problem assessment by putting the patient at the centre of the tests.

Advocate: This is the responsibility of the nurse. Works on helping handle things like insurance and covering of medical bills.

Manager: handle health care cases

Educator: Giving the relevant information to at-home patients and giving them useful information within short periods of time. This is effective when thorough training on the situation is not possible

27 SPIKES Protocol for Delivering Bad News

Even though it is your work to make things better and nurse patients back to health, you sometimes are entitled with the responsibility of passing on bad news. Before making the news know, you have to ensure that you go through a set of steps to prepare both you and the recipient for the bad news. SPIKES are the mnemonic you need to remember what to do.

1: S- Set the interview on your patient: organize for a good place and time to meet with the person.

2: P- Perception of your assessment: understand the recipient temperament. This will determine how he/she might perceive the news.

3: I- Invitation of the right interviewee: Know the right people who can be invited to the interview.

4: K- Knowledge and information: Have a complete and comprehensive layout of the information. You do not have to make pauses and confirmation or make wrong statements as this will increase anxiety.

5: E- Emotions and empathy: Take care of the recipients emotional needs by being sympathetic and empathetic.

Step 6: S- Strategize and summarize: Make the meeting as short as possible.

28 Cyanotic Defects 4 T's

This refers to a set of heart problems that are cognitive. The will affect the flow of blood in the body sometimes leading to anemic like conditions and loss of oxygen supply to the rest of the body. Commons signs to condition will include clubbing, crying, tachypnea and tachycardia. The 4 T's represent different types of the condition.

Tetralogy of Fallot: These children will have blue-tinged skin and cyanotic. The condition makes oxygen poor blood to leave the heart.

Truncus Arteriosus: Only one large blood vessel leaves the heart instead of two. Also, lower and upper chamber do not have the separating walls hence oxygenated and deoxygenated blood mixes up.

Transposition of great arteries: It is not common. The two arteries leaving the heart are transposed meaning one part of the body will not get as enough oxygenated blood as it needs

Tricuspid Atresia: The valves between the two heart chamber not formed. Blood cannot flow through the heart to lungs effectively.

Some of these conditions can be handled by behavioral mitigation of the symptoms. Others need to be operated on as soon as possible.

29 Psychiatric assessment

Even though psychiatrist assessment might be the work of a doctor, you sometimes have to edit your service delivery based on what you observe. Always Send Mail Through the Post Office will help you remember the diagnosis steps.

Appearance: the general look and appearance of the patient at first glance

Speech: how the patient is talking and responding to your questions

Memory/mood: some problems will affect your memory, others mood. Observe these aspects of the patient.

Thoughts: What the patient thinks about his condition could help you make an elaborate inference of what he or she is actually going through.

Perception: Your perception of the patient's condition and different body language signs he or she passes.

Orientation: How the patient is well versed with his or her immediate surroundings.

Part 6. AIDS and HIV Acronyms and Mnemonics

30 HIV Prevention: you must Wrap, Glove and Shoot

WRAP it, simply means the use of condom in patients who are engaged with sexual intercourse with other. Other than just encouraging the use of the condom, also teach the person how to use the condom appropriately.

GLOVE, people who have contacts with patient who happened to have HIV need to use gloves every time they are having contact with the patient. This forms protection to the second most common way of HIV/AIDS transmission.

Don't SHOOT up (intravenous drug users must not share needles) This is advice for drug users. It focuses on the common sharing piercing material problem that leads to transmission of the disease.

31 HIV Transmission: Vertical VS Horizontal

Vertical: from mother to infant during birth. This is so since a baby is come up in vertical way from your pelvis.

Horizontal: this is through body fluid and as well as in having sexual intercourse. Sexual intercourse mostly happens in horizontal positions.

32 HIV and AIDS Risk Assessment: AIDS

Afraid of exposure to the virus

Intravenous drug use

Diagnostic features of HIV infections; e.g.: reoccurring thrush infections) to validate or nullify the fear

Sexual behaviors that put the patient in risk of sex should hint towards the need for a test.

33 HIV Body Fluid Transmission: BBB

This is perfect for identifying the different bodily fluids that can lead to the transmission of the HIV virus from one person to another.

Blood

Bodily fluids when having sex

Breast milk

34 HIV Drugs: RIP

RALFSINA are said to be the Inhibitors of Protease or the inhibitors of Protease

RALFSINA: simply means the Ritonavir, Amprenavir, Lopinavir, Fosamprenavir, Saquinavir, Indinavir, Nelfinavir, Atazanavir

There are a couple of drugs used to handle the HIV. They all exist in batches and it is up to you to keep the right medication groups together in your mind with these acronyms.

Conclusion

There are many medical conditions that any professional nurse must have in mind in order to carry out his or her duties efficiently. While some of the most common and frequently occurring conditions will sink into mind faster, sometimes, you have to get some memory aids to help you remember the things you will not be handling on a daily basis.

Thank You Page

I want to personally thank you for reading my book. I hope you found information in this book useful and I would be very grateful if you could leave your honest review about this book. I certainly want to thank you in advance for doing this.

If you have the time, you can check my other books too.